Empowering Wellness

A Comprehensive Guide to Diabetes Management

Copyright

Preface

Living with diabetes is a journey filled with challenges, triumphs, and opportunities for growth. As healthcare professionals dedicated to supporting individuals with diabetes, we recognize the importance of providing comprehensive education and resources to empower individuals in managing their condition effectively. This course serves as a testament to our commitment to promoting holistic health and wellness for individuals living with diabetes. The content presented in this course is grounded In the latest research, clinical guidelines, and best practices in diabetes care. Our aim is to equip participants with the knowledge, skills, and confidence to navigate the complexities of diabetes management with resilience and grace. Through a blend of evidence-based information, practical tips, and interactive learning experiences, we strive to empower individuals to take control of their health and achieve optimal well-being.

We extend our gratitude to the individuals living with diabetes who generously shared their experiences and insights, as well as to the healthcare professionals and researchers whose dedication and expertise have informed the development of this book. It is our sincere hope that this resource will serve as a valuable companion on your journey to living well with diabetes.

Together, let us embark on this journey of discovery, learning, and empowerment, as we strive towards a future where every individual with diabetes can thrive and flourish.

Table of Contents

Introduction

Living with diabetes comes with special problems that call for a multimodal approach to care. In order to live well with diabetes, people need to arm themselves with information and skills related to the disease, including how to manage it through lifestyle modifications and treatment options. This extensive course covers important subjects like medication administration, stress management, exercise, diet, and preventive measures in an effort to provide a comprehensive approach to diabetes care. Through the provision of evidence-based strategies and useful tools, this course aims to assist individuals in reaching their best health outcomes and improving their overall quality of life.

Understanding Diabetes

Millions of people worldwide suffer with diabetes, a chronic illness that is frequently misdiagnosed. This page explores the complexities of diabetes, illuminating its forms, origins, signs, and possible side effects.

Types of Diabetes

There are various types of diabetes, such as

Type 1, _Type 2_, and _gestational diabetes_.

 Type 1 diabetes is usually diagnosed in childhood and is caused by the body's inability to make insulin.

Type 2 diabetes is more common in adults and is frequently linked to lifestyle variables like diet and exercise.

gestational diabetes occurs during pregnancy which needs to be carefully managed to prevent complications for the mother and the unborn child.

It is essential to comprehend diabetes symptoms in order to recognize and treat the condition early. Increased thirst, frequent urination, unexplained weight loss, exhaustion, and blurred eyesight are some of these. Diabetes can cause major side effects like heart disease, renal failure, and nerve damage if it is not controlled.

By dispelling misconceptions about diabetes and increasing knowledge, we enable people to identify its symptoms, get the right medical attention, and take proactive measures to manage it well.

Nutrition's Impact on Diabetes Treatment

Blood sugar regulation, weight control, and general well-being are all greatly influenced by nutrition, which is also essential for managing diabetes. We discuss the fundamentals of a diabetes-friendly diet in this post and offer helpful hints for organising meals and maintaining a healthy diet.

The control of carbohydrates is essential to diabetes diet. Blood sugar levels are directly impacted by carbohydrates, therefore it's critical to watch consumption and make informed decisions. To maintain stable blood glucose levels throughout the day, moderate meal sizes and prioritise healthy grains, fruits, vegetables, and lean proteins.

Take into account the food's glycemic index (GI), which rates the pace at which carbs elevate blood sugar. Choose low-GI foods to avoid blood glucose spikes and crashes. Including a variety of fats, proteins, and carbohydrates in meals can help to further encourage fullness and discourage overindulging.

Those with diabetes can optimise their health and vitality, laying the groundwork for long-term wellness and disease control, by embracing a balanced and attentive approach to eating.

The Influence of Exercise on Diabetes Management

With so many advantages for emotional and physical well-being, exercise is a powerful ally in the fight against diabetes. In this piece, we examine how regular exercise can improve blood sugar regulation, weight control, and general wellbeing.

Walking, swimming, or cycling are

examples of aerobic exercises that can help reduce blood sugar and increase insulin sensitivity. Conversely, strength training activities improve metabolic function and muscle mass, which help with long-term glucose control and weight maintenance.

Beyond its physiological benefits, exercise is essential for lowering stress and improving mood, two things that can have a significant influence on the treatment of diabetes. People with diabetes can lower their risk of complications and live better lives by making regular physical activity a part of their daily routine.

Effective diabetes care revolves around enabling people to adopt an active lifestyle, which provides a route to long-term health, resilience, and energy.

Managing Diabetes Medication and Insulin Therapy

Medication and insulin therapy are important parts of the treatment plan for many diabetic patients. We give a summary of the many drugs that are available, their modes of action, and factors to take into account when managing insulin in this article.

Different strategies are used by diabetic drugs to lower blood sugar: either by boosting insulin sensitivity, decreasing intestinal glucose absorption, or increasing insulin synthesis. People should collaborate closely with their healthcare providers to identify the best pharmaceutical regimen for them, taking into account their unique needs and current state of health.

Insulin therapy may be required in cases of advanced Type 2 diabetes or Type 1 diabetes in order to maintain ideal blood glucose control. For safe and efficient administration, it is crucial to comprehend insulin kinds, administration methods, and dosage modifications. Because continuous glucose monitoring (CGM) devices provide real-time input on blood sugar levels, they can also help with insulin dosing decisions.

People may make educated decisions about their treatment options and collaborate with their healthcare team to achieve optimal health outcomes by understanding diabetes drugs and insulin therapy.

The Significance of Blood Glucose Control in Diabetes Treatment

A key component of managing diabetes is routine blood glucose monitoring, which offers important information about general health and the efficacy of therapy. This post examines the importance of blood glucose monitoring and provides helpful advice for maximising self-care.

People can keep track of how their bodies react to diet, exercise, medications, and other circumstances by monitoring their blood sugar levels. Through the establishment of goal ranges and the regular monitoring of blood glucose levels throughout the day, patients can discern patterns, discern trends, and advise any necessary modifications to their treatment regimen.

Traditional glucose metres, continuous glucose monitors (CGMs), and flash glucose monitoring systems are just a few of the monitoring tools that are available. To accommodate varying tastes and lifestyles, these tools provide a variety of features and functionalities.

Providing people with the information and abilities to properly check their blood glucose levels is essential to attaining the best possible diabetes care and lowering the risk of complications.

Self-monitoring is a path towards wellbeing and vitality that people can take control of by adopting regular habits

Stress Reduction Techniques for Diabetes Wellbeing

Stress management is essential to preserving general well-being because managing diabetes can be difficult. In this piece, we examine the complex connections among stress, diabetes, and mental health while providing doable methods for developing inner calm and resilience.

Stress can have a substantial effect on blood sugar levels by inducing hormonal reactions that may compromise glucose regulation and insulin sensitivity. In addition, poor coping mechanisms like emotional eating and skipping self-care rituals may be influenced by chronic stress.

Creating efficient stress-reduction strategies is crucial to reducing these impacts and advancing holistic health. Deep breathing exercises, yoga, and meditation are examples of mindfulness techniques that can assist people in developing present-moment awareness and lowering their stress levels.

In addition, developing a robust support system and getting expert advice through counselling or therapy can be quite helpful in managing the psychological effects of diabetes. People with diabetes are better able to handle the ups and downs of life with greater resilience and grace when they prioritise self-care and mental health.

How Sleep Affects Diabetes Management

It is impossible to overestimate the significance of getting enough good sleep for managing diabetes and for maintaining general health and wellbeing. In this piece, we examine the complex connection between diabetes and sleep, providing information on how improving sleep hygiene might enhance blood sugar regulation and general health.

An increase in insulin resistance and raised blood sugar levels can result from poor sleep patterns that disturb hormonal balance and impede glucose metabolism, such as irregular sleep schedules, sleep deprivation, or sleep disorders like sleep apnea. On the other hand, putting restorative sleep first can improve blood glucose management and insulin sensitivity.

Maintaining a regular sleep schedule, establishing a calming bedtime ritual, enhancing the conditions of the sleep environment, and minimising exposure to stimulating activities or devices before bedtime are easy ways to improve sleep hygiene. To address sleep-related concerns and optimise diabetes control, it is imperative that patients with underlying sleep disturbances seek medical examination and treatment.

People can prioritise sleep as a crucial part of their self-care routine after realising the important connection between sleep and diabetes, which will promote better health and a higher standard of living.

Methods to Avoid Complications from Diabetes

The key to managing diabetes effectively is preventing complications, which highlights the significance of taking preventative actions to protect long-term health. In this post, we'll look at methods for reducing problems from diabetes and encouraging overall wellbeing.

The heart, kidneys, eyes, nerves, and other organs and systems in the body are among those that might be impacted by diabetes problems. It is essential to keep blood pressure, cholesterol, and blood sugar within target ranges in order to lower the risk of consequences such renal disease, neuropathy, retinopathy, and cardiovascular disease.

Diet, exercise, and stress reduction are examples of lifestyle variables that are important in averting problems and enhancing general health. A balanced diet high in fruits, vegetables, whole grains, and lean proteins, together with frequent exercise and stress management practices, can help people stay as healthy as possible and lessen the negative effects of diabetes on their bodies.

Self-monitoring techniques, tests, and routine medical checkups are critical for early diagnosis and management, enabling people to handle possible issues before they worsen. People with diabetes can reduce their risk of complications and live longer by managing their diabetes proactively and giving preventive treatment first priority.

Handling Diabetes Support Communities

Coping with diabetes can be quite demanding at times, but you don't have to do it by yourself. In order to successfully traverse the difficulties of managing diabetes, we discuss in this article the significance of reaching out for assistance and making connections with resources.

There are many different kinds of support networks, such as those made up of friends, family, medical professionals, support groups, internet forums, and advocacy groups. These networks provide people with diabetes with priceless tools, support, and empathy, enabling them to feel empowered and part of a community.

Diabetes support networks offer chances for exchanging experiences and insights, educational materials, and practical guidance in addition to emotional support. Support networks provide an abundance of information and companionship, whether one is looking for guidance on controlling blood sugar levels, handling the psychological effects of diabetes, or navigating healthcare institutions.

People with diabetes can discover hope, resiliency, and strength in the face of adversity by connecting with others who have experienced similar things. Creating connections within the diabetic community helps people feel like they belong and are not alone, which gives them the confidence to succeed in spite of any challenges they may face.

Establishing Objectives for Diabetes Care

One effective strategy for enabling people with diabetes to take charge of their health and well-being is goal-setting. In this piece, we examine the significance of goal-setting and action planning in the management of diabetes, providing doable tactics for attaining significant results.

Setting realistic, attainable goals and recognising areas for development are the first steps in creating an effective goal-setting strategy. Setting definite, well-defined goals provide direction and incentive for action, whether the aim is stress management, weight loss, physical activity increase, or blood sugar control.

By dividing goals into more manageable chunks, people can get beyond obstacles and maintain focus on their goals. Establishing deadlines and monitoring results along the way encourage positive behaviour and momentum towards long-term health objectives by allowing for modifications and celebrating accomplishments.

Setting goals that are Specific, Measurable, Achievable, Relevant, and Time-bound (SMART) guarantees accountability and clarity and raises the probability of success. People can stay on course to achieve optimal health outcomes by regularly reviewing and reflecting on their objectives and action plans and making necessary adjustments to their tactics.

Through the utilisation of goal setting and action planning, people with diabetes can develop a heightened sense of agency, resilience, and empowerment in the management of their illness, ultimately realising their maximum potential for optimal health and well-being.